HEALING POWER IN YOUR HOME

Master herbalist David Hoffmann presents a basic collection of 21 therapeutically valuable herbs and explains how they can help in dealing with everyday health problems from digestive upsets to migraines and wound healing. You'll also find out how to prepare and store herbal remedies and how to be sure of getting the best-quality herbs for your money.

ABOUT THE AUTHOR

David Hoffmann is a medical herbalist and Director of the California School of Herbal Studies in Forestville. He has written, lectured and appeared on TV and radio extensively, and his work has been the subject of a TV documentary. He has written four books on herbal and health topics, and has studied herbal lore in Europe, the Near East and Asia.

YOUR HERBAL HOME MEDICINE CHEST

DAVID HOFFMANN, B.Sc., M.N.I.M.H.

Keats Publishing, Inc. New Canaan, Connecticut

Your Herbal Home Medicine Chest is not intended as medical advice. Its intention is solely informational and educational. Please consult a medical or health professional should the need for one be indicated.

YOUR HERBAL HOME MEDICINE CHEST

Copyright © 1989 by David Hoffmann

All rights reserved

No part of this book may be copied or reproduced in any form without the written consent of the publisher.

ISBN: 0-87983-508-7
Printed in the United States of America

The Self-Care Health Library is published by
Keats Publishing, Inc.
27 Pine Street (Box 876)
New Canaan, Connecticut 06840

CONTENTS

	Page
An Herbal Medicine Chest for the Home	7
Healing with the Medicine Chest	11
Remedies for the Medicine Chest	20
The Preparation of Herbs	28
Herbal Next Steps	30
Bibliography	31
References	32

AN HERBAL MEDICINE CHEST FOR THE HOME

This booklet is designed to reintroduce the simple and effective art of home herbalism. The gift of healing plants is a birthright of all people, not simply those we call experts. Herbalism is an ancient art that has thrived in all cultures of the world, in all historical periods, a constant and vital thread in human life. Herbal knowledge still persists, although the traditional wisdom of the herbalist is difficult to find. This little book will help home herbalists empower themselves with the skills and knowledge of this wonderful field, though it will not replace more detailed herbals.

The Healing Potential of Herbal Remedies

Herbal medicine has a breadth of use as wide as any form of medicine. Herbs may be used for any condition that is medically treatable. This is not claiming that herbalism is a cure-all or panacea for the ills of humanity, but that interaction of plant activity with human physiology offers the potential for facilitating the healing process at any time in any situation.

Herbs are simple, safe and effective remedies that are ideal as part of home self-help treatments. You do not need a professionally trained medical herbalist to use plant remedies for the minor ills that abound in family life, but more serious problems do call for the skills of a trained professional.

The health and wholeness of ourselves and those we love is a vital concern, but one often handed into someone else's care. In these times of medical complexity and confusion, society has come to depend upon the expert. The benefits of our specialized health care system have been paid for in many ways, one being a loss of personal responsibility for health and well-being. The skills of health care workers are lifesaving, but society has perhaps gone too far in empowering professional élites at the expense of self-help.

A new understanding of health is appearing. This change in attitude and approach is integral to what is often referred to as Holistic Medicine, and is part of a whole shift in the way we see ourselves, our place in the wider world, and the issues that effect us. The World Health Organization's definition has a simplicity which highlights its profound relevance:

> Health is more than simply the absence of illness, it is an active state of physical emotional, mental and social well-being.

A wonderful expression of the perspectives of holistic medicine! This approach starts from the assumption that health is a positive and active state, that is an inherent characteristic of whole and integrated human beings. From a holistic standpoint, a person is not a patient with a disease syndrome but a whole being. This wholeness requires that therapists appreciate the mental, emotional, spiritual and social aspects of their patients' lives as well as the physical. A holistic practitioner, of whatever specific therapy, has a deep respect for the individual's capacity for self-healing, allowing a relationship of active partners in the healing process, rather than expert and passive recipient.

Herbalism fits well into holistic medicine. It is a healing technique that is fundamentally in tune with nature. It has been described as ecological healing as it is because of our shared ecological and evolutionary heritage with the plant kingdom that herbal remedies work.

How to Select a Remedy

There are well over two thousand plants used in herbal medicine in the western world, and the planet-wide list is far longer. So what can you realistically provide in the home?

Selecting remedies to use and to get to know is the first step. One way of doing this is to read through a herbal from a to z (Abscess root to Zedoary!) until you find just what you need. This takes a lot of time, and although it may be fun, it won't help the illness. Or you can use a source book that lists conditions and describes herbal treatments. This is fine but limiting, as it means doing what the author tells you to do for a particular ailment, rather than taking into account that each sick person is unique and not simply a disease host.

The medical herbalist used a model that enables a prescription to be formulated that addresses the needs of the whole person. It is based upon:

- herbal actions
- system affinity
- specific remedies for the illness
- herbal biochemistry
- intuition

Herbal actions describe the ways in which the remedy affects human physiology. Plants have a direct impact on physiological activity, and by knowing what body process you want to help or heal, you can select the appropriate action. These actions are described in the next section, "Healing with the Medicine Chest."

Some herbs show an affinity for certain organs or body systems. They work as specific tonics or nutrients for the areas involved. Herbs can be used freely and safely as part of one's lifestyle without thinking of them as "medicines." They are at their best when used to nurture health and vitality, thus preventing health problems from arising. During illness the system affinity herbs will enhance the general health of the organ or system involved when combined with remedies selected for their actions. They are especially useful where a tendency towards illness is recognized but no overt disease is present. Using herbs in this way opens the possibility of overcoming a weakness that could lead to disease later in life.

The wealth of herbal knowledge that has been garnered over many generations abounds in plants that are traditionally specific in the treatment of certain diseases or symptoms. Holistic healing goes beyond symptomatic therapy, but this knowledge deserves great respect. Knowledge of specific remedies can add much to a formula based on appropriate actions and system support.

Increasing attention is being given to the biochemistry of herbal active ingredients. This has led to the development of many lifesaving drugs, but is very limited as an approach to using whole plants. It will not be explored in this book.

There is a flowering of intuitive rapport between herbalist and the plants. Intuition has a special role to play in healing, and the unique relationship between plant and person augments it.

The home herbalist can follow a similar model, making it possible to treat most everyday health problems. Using the ideas of actions and system affinity, a small number of remedies can be selected to provide a range of therapeutic possibilities. The rest of this book will explore them.

Stocking the Medicine Chest

It is fairly easy to stock a small herbal medicine chest which will fulfill most day-to-day needs. The herbs on the following list possess among them all the main actions, and there are some specifics as well. Become thoroughly familiar with these plants, and use them with discretion. They may be stored as tinctures (alcohol solutions), tablets or dried herbs.

Boneset	Calendula	Chamomile
Dandelion	Devil's claw	Echinacea
Elecampane	Feverfew	Ginkgo
Golden seal	Hawthorn	Linden flower
Marshmallow	Meadowsweet	Milk thistle
Nettles	St. John's wort	Siberian ginseng
Uva-ursi	Valerian	

In addition to these medicinal herbs, there are the wonderful culinary herbs and spices that have valuable healing properties, but there is not room to go into them here. John Heinerman's *Complete Book of Spices* (Keats Publishing), treats this topic thoroughly.

Herb Quality

There are two main obstacles to overcome in ensuring a good experience of herbal medicine. This first is an ill-informed remedy selection, and the second is using herbs of low quality. It is not surprising that herbal therapy has a reputation of working slowly if at all! Reliability of herbal products is a fundamental issue. With the ever-growing array of herbal products, simply being herbal is not enough—the quality of the herb is all-important.

When choosing remedies there are certain guidelines that will help in the face of the confusing range of products available. At first glance it may seem that a plant is a plant and that is all there is to it. I'm afraid not! Unless you are picking your own fresh herbs, they will have been through a number of stages of drying and preparing. At each one of these steps skilled care must be taken to ensure that the healing activity of the plant is maintained, if possible enhanced. It is vital to select products manufactured with such care.

An excellent guideline is standardization of products on internationally recognized principles. Such standards help ensure that the healing quality of the plant is going to be maintained in the manufactured product. Throughout Europe, herbal medicine is a well-respected component of health care, and a wealth of information on quality control and standards is available, especially in Germany and Britain. Because of the extensive research needed to establish standardization of each plant, not all the herbs in our medicine chest are currently standardized. One company, Yerba Prima Botanicals, is leading the way in making available standardized herbs based on the latest research.

To be sure of getting a high-quality product, check the label for the standardized component; for instance, Yerba Prima's golden seal root is standardized at 5% alkaloids, and is so labeled. In the section on individual remedies, the appropriate standardizing component is listed, when there is one.

In practice, a specific constituent or group of constituents acts as markers whose levels are used as a standard for assessing quality. These are measured using chromatography, a basic laboratory procedure that is the established technique used in official pharmacopoeias world wide. The herb industry would do a great service to the whole field of health care if it used and adhered to these pharmacopeial standards. Complete standardization is impossible, due to the complexity and diversity of plants, and it may in any case not be the levels of measured constituents that influences the biological activity of the whole plant. There is a synergistic interaction between all the components, both "active" and "inert," that creates an effect that is more than simply the sum of the separate ingredients activity. Standardization of herbal products using certain constituents as markers does not discard the plant in favor of active ingredients, but it ensures a maintenance of the miraculous wholeness offered by nature for our health and well-being.

Using standardized remedies assures that you will get good-quality herbs that have been correctly identified and grown, collected and dried properly. You will also not need as large doses as otherwise, since useful levels of active substances will be present with a relatively small amount of the plant. This makes it more convenient and reduces costs.

HEALING WITH THE MEDICINE CHEST

From the rich traditional roots of herbalism has come the knowledge of specific remedies for specific symptoms and diseases. This wealth of knowledge, based on generations of experience, provides the modern herbalist with a solid foundation from which to embrace the insights of science and contribute much to the new approaches of holistic medicine.

However, for those wanting to use herbs in their own health care, this abundance is overpowering! The herbs that are discussed here can provide a whole spectrum of possibilities if their actions are compared and combined, allowing most common problems to be tackled by the beginner herbalist.

Most of the important actions of herbs are performed by even the comparatively few herbs discussed in this book. Here is a brief description of these actions and some of the herbs which perform them.

Adaptogen: increasing resistance to stress
  Siberian ginseng

Alterative: restoring proper bodily function
  Dandelion, echinacea, garlic, nettles

Analgesic: relieving pain
  Devil's claw, meadowsweet, valerian

Antacid: relieving stomach acidity and distress
  Meadowsweet

Anticatarrhal: removing excess mucus in sinus and other areas
  Boneset, devil's claw, echinacea, garlic, golden seal

Anti-inflammatory: soothing tissue inflammation
  Calendula, chamomile, devil's claw, feverfew, meadowsweet, St. John's wort

Antimicrobial: resisting pathogenic microorganisms, usually by strengthening the immune system
  Calendula, chamomile, echinacea, elecampane, garlic, uva-ursi

Antispasmodic: easing muscular cramp and sometimes psychological tension
  Boneset, chamomile, garlic, linden flowers, valerian

Aperient: mildly laxative
  Boneset

Astringent: binding to skin and mucous tissue, reducing irritation and inflammation, protecting against infection
  Golden seal, meadowsweet, nettles, St. John's wort

Bitter: stimulating to appetite, to digestion, to liver function
  Chamomile, dandelion, feverfew, golden seal

Carminative: stimulating and soothing to the digestive system, removing gas
  Chamomile, meadowsweet, linden flowers, valerian
Cardiac tonic: having a beneficial effect on the heart
  Hawthorn
Cholagogue: promoting bile flow
  Calendula, dandelion root, garlic
Demulcent: reducing irritation and protecting inflamed tissue through high mucilage content
  Marshmallow, milk thistle
Diaphoretic: promoting sweating and capillary dilation
  Boneset, elecampane, garlic, linden flowers, peppermint
Diuretic: increasing the secretion and elimination of urine
  Boneset, dandelion, linden flowers, marshmallow, meadowsweet, uva-ursi
Emmenagogue: normalizing and toning the female reproductive system
  Calendula
Emollient: soothing, softening
  Marshmallow
Expectorant: stimulating the removal of mucus from the lungs; in general, a tonic for the respiratory system
  Elecampane, marshmallow
Hepatic: strengthening and toning the liver
  Garlic, dandelion, golden seal, milk thistle
Galactagogue: promoting secretion of milk
  Milk thistle
Hypotensive: lowering abnormally high blood pressure
  Garlic, hawthorn, linden flowers, valerian
Laxative: stimulating to bowel action
  Boneset, golden seal
Nervine: acting beneficially on the nervous system, as either tonics, relaxants or stimulants
  Calendula, chamomile, linden flowers, St. John's wort, valerian
Sedative: promoting sleep
  Valerian
Tonic: nuturing and enlivening
  Calendula, chamomile, echinacea, garlic, golden seal, hawthorn, nettles
Vasodilator: expanding blood vessels
  Feverfew, ginkgo, Siberian ginseng
Vulnerary: promoting healing of wounds and ulcers
  Calendula, marshmallow, St. John's wort

Through applying this basic model of using herbal action to address the physiological need of the individual, many health problems can be treated with even this small number of remedies. Treatments for the conditions discussed next will demonstrate the potentials for using these, but a more comprehensive herbal should be consulted for in-depth information or problems not covered here.

Maintaining Health

A number of steps can be taken to nurture the health that even the most frail person is blessed with. This involves not only nurturing the body but caring for emotions and thoughts with the same depth of attention. To be healthy we must be whole.

• Experience the embrace of nature, through herbs as well as walks or even hugging a tree. Smile!
• Eat a healthy balanced diet
• Ensure good elimination
• Build any therapeutic program undertaken around gentle tonic herbs, and not simply the strong remedies that focus on symptoms.
• Find a coping strategy for stress and the challenges of life that works for you.
• Nurture any physical weakness. This may be due to past illness, accident or current problems. Use remedies to fortify that part of the body or body function. Here are examples of remedies that have a toning effect on the systems of the body and may safely be used over extended periods of time. They are not all described in this book.

Circulatory system	Hawthorn
Respiratory system	Elecampane
Digestive system	Chamomile
Nervous system	Skullcap
Skin	Nettles
Muscular and skeletal system	Celery seed
Reproductive system	Raspberry leaves
Urinary system	Buchu

Cleansing and Detoxification

The four primary pathways of elimination are the digestive system, kidneys, lungs and the skin. Each makes major contribution and if one is not functioning well because of illness, the others carry an extra load. The digestive system cleanses via the colon and through the detoxification and natural laxative work of the liver. The use of strong herbal laxatives to empty the bowel is to be avoided, as they can lead to dependency. The best way to promote bowel cleansing is via the liver, as with the use of dandelion, and dietary fiber.

The kidneys cleanse the blood and excrete waste in the urine. Herbal diuretics such as dandelion, nettles and uva-ursi help this process. The skin eliminates waste in sweat, which is helped by diaphoretic remedies such as boneset and linden flowers.

A detoxification program uses remedies that focus on these pathways while aiding any organs that are under special pressure. This will vary with each unique individual, and the specifics go beyond the scope of this book. Please refer to *The Herbal Handbook* by David Hoffmann. A useful combination would be golden seal, nettles and dandelion. As the tea would have an unpleasant taste, a combination of tinctures or tablets would be best. This should be taken along with a natural fiber colon cleansing program as described by Dr. Jeffrey Bland in an excellent book about the Yerba Prima program.[1]

Infections and Immunity

Ensuring a vibrant immune system involves taking care of the whole person. Through diet, exercise and safe medicine when needed, a healthy body will provide a firm foundation for immunity. Feelings have a direct impact upon immune response, highlighting the need for emotional well-being.

A number of different levels can be supported herbally. Nature provides a wealth of plants to support resistance to disease. Antimicrobial herbs such as echinacea, calendula, golden seal and garlic can prevent and treat infection. In small amounts taken regularly they boost resistance, or larger doses combat specific infections. Diaphoretics such as boneset, linden flowers, cayenne and ginger also help.

Stress must be treated, as it has a direct impact on immunity. The more pressure endured, the more battering the immune system sustains. In addition to working with a stress management program, use adaptogenic herbs such as Siberian ginseng.

Colds and Flu

A tendency to frequent colds is the body's hint that the immune system needs help. Echinacea, golden seal and garlic help prevent colds.

To treat an infection once started, address the symptoms and support the body's fight against the virus. Perhaps the best is the diaphoretic boneset, especially if there is a fever. Drinking a hot infusion will often make life bearable in even the worst cases of flu. Chamomile, linden flower and peppermint tea will have a similar effect—and, while not as strong, they do taste a lot better! The bitter taste of boneset is one of its therapeutic trademarks, but not a quality most people relish.

Do not inhibit nasal congestion with anticatarrhal drugs, as this is a normal body response to infection. Herbal anticatarrhals work in a very different and safer way. Chamomile, peppermint or boneset will relieve much of the symptomatic discomfort. Golden seal will speed the healing, as will raw garlic or garlic oil capsules.

To help the immune system use antimicrobial herbs such as echinacea and golden seal and the tonic nettle. These may be combined in capsules, or as tinctures. Garlic in food or in oil capsules would be most beneficial.

Coughs

A cough is an important sign, and should not be simply suppressed. Any long-standing or intransigent coughing should receive professional attention. Home treatment is safe and effective for minor coughs of short duration or associated with mild infections, but if in doubt seek skilled advice.

Expectorant remedies help get rid of phlegm in the lungs, but also soothe irritation and reduce the cough reflex. Elecampane is safe and effective for both children and adults. Use as an infusion at least 3 times a day as long as the symptoms remain. If there is a dry, irritating cough, use a demulcent such as marshmallow leaves to soothe the inflamed membranes. There are many effective kitchen remedies for cough. Slice an onion into a deep bowl and cover in honey and let stand overnight. Strain off the mixture of juice and honey. This makes a simple cough elixir. Take a dessertspoon 4 or 5 times a day.

Hayfever

Hayfever responds differently with each person, so try different approaches until the right one is found. The only specific herb is a Chinese plant that is not in our medicine chest called Ma Huang (*Ephedra sinica*). It is a herb to have around if hayfever is a problem. Apart from Ma Huang, the most effective approach is to address the symptoms that are present. Anticatarrhal herbs will ease the runny nose. Try golden seal, chamomile or boneset. For dry and irritating eyes make a wash of chamomile, or simply apply a thin fresh slice of cucumber to the closed eyes. The alterative remedies may help in easing the underlying sensitivity. Regular nettle tea will help. Raw garlic in honey has been used traditionally for the relief of symptoms.

Heart Disease and High Blood Pressure

Although plant medicines offer much for the treatment of heart disease, this is an area where professional advice is essential. Some herbs have a potent and direct impact upon the heart itself, such as foxglove, and form the basis of drug therapy for heart failure. These can be lifesaving remedies, but must be prescribed by skilled practitioners, and so are not included in the home medicine chest. The herbs suggested in this booklet are safe and gentle cardiac tonics, ideal as preventive support. They have a significant long-term effect in helping to reduce cholesterol and gently opening coronary arteries to increase blood flow to the heart. Clinical studies have shown hawthorn to have a coronary artery-dilating effect, and garlic to have a persistent cholesterol-lowering effect; other herbs beneficial to the heart are linden flowers, motherwort, cramp bark, yarrow and rosemary. The nervines chamomile and valerian will help reduce stress, usually a contributor to heart problems, and dandelion's diuretic properties will relieve water retention.

Stress is also often involved in high blood pressure, as is diet; reducing animal fats and salt and increasing fruits and vegetables is known to be helpful. A clove of garlic—raw—a day will help normalize blood pressure; so will an infusion of hawthorn berries twice a day. Linden flowers added to the hawthorn infusion will strengthen the effect.

Circulation and Varicose Veins

Cayenne or ginger are herbs which will stimulate blood circulation; those that strengthen and dilate the vessels include hawthorn and linden flowers. Ginkgo promotes capillary circulation, relieving leg pain and increasing the capacity for walking.

For varicose veins, a tea made from equal parts of hawthorn, linden flowers and nettles will strengthen the blood vessel walls over time. Tablets of the herbs may be used instead. A wash of calendula will ease any inflammation and reduce the discomfort.

Arthritis

Arthritis is a general term for approximately 100 diseases that produce either inflammation of connective tissues, particularly in joints, or noninflammatory degeneration of these tissues. Herbal medicine is uniquely appropriate for these problems, as it works with the whole body, promoting an improvement of the condition while it alleviates pain and discomfort. The alterative herbs form the basis of treatment, helping the body remove toxins and waste that act as a focus for illness. Echinacea, nettles and dandelion work in this way. The diuretic action of dandelion helps flush the body. The nervines valerian, linden flowers and chamomile may be used to relax muscle tension and ease joint tightness. Circulatory stimulants such as cayenne, ginger, and mustard increase blood flow to both muscles and bones, increasing availability of nutrients and promoting removal of waste. Anti-inflammatory herbs, such as meadowsweet, devil's claw and feverfew will ease pain and discomfort.

Warming remedies will help circulation and ease pain locally if applied as plasters or poultices. (See the section on preparation of herbs.) Mustard or cayenne are very effective if used in moderation. A cabbage poultice is a traditional remedy in France.

Diarrhea and Constipation

Diarrhea is usually the natural response to infection or irritation of some part of the digestive tract. As long as the diarrhea is not due to some more pressing medical problem, it is best to let the condition run its course, replacing lost fluids and electrolytes by drinking a solution of warm water and honey. If the problem persists, use an astringent such as nettle. If nothing else is available, use very strong black tea. Echinacea or garlic will help combat any infection that might be present, and chamomile will settle feelings of nausea.

The best approach to constipation is a high-fiber diet and adequate exercise. A fiber-based colon cleansing program is the most effective and safe treatment. This is described in another book in this series.[2] Strong herbal laxatives such as senna or cascara should be avoided, but the gentle effects of dandelion are fine.

Ulcers

Using plants having demulcent, antacid, astringent and vulnerary actions makes it possible to bring about a rapid and complete healing of most ulcers. Marshmallow, calendula, meadowsweet, chamomile and golden seal are examples of such remedies.

Reducing stress through changes in lifestyle, relaxation, and exercise combined with herbal relaxing nervines is also important. An infusion of chamomile, linden flowers or valerian will help. For the ulcer itself drink an infusion 3 times a day, using a teaspoon of a mixture containing 1 part chamomile, 1 part meadowsweet and 2 parts marshmallow root. When the discomfort has subsided, add 1 part golden seal to the mixture. Combining high-quality tablets will have the same results.

The Liver

Another area of therapy that is well suited for herbal treatment is that of liver damage. The liver serves the body in a wide range of vital functions. It is able to regenerate itself after being injured or diseased, but if a disease progresses beyond the tissues' capacity to regenerate new cells, the body's entire metabolism is severely affected.

With hepatic remedies such as golden seal, dandelion and milk thistle in our medicine chest, it is possible to deal with conditions requiring gentle liver stimulation or even to treat profound liver disease.

As with most claims made by the medical herbalist, pharmacological and clinical research is starting to support traditional experience and provide a chemical insight into the mechanisms involved. A good example is the milk thistle. Historically this herb has been used in Europe as a liver tonic and is now used in a whole range of liver and gall bladder conditions including hepatitis and cirrhosis. It may also have value in the treatment of chronic uterine problems. A wealth of research done in Germany is revealing exciting data about reversal of toxic liver damage as well as protection from potential liver toxins.[3]

The Nervous System

All of the many herbal nervines effect body symptoms as well as the mind. An example is motherwort, a nervine used in treating anxiety and tension that also has specific affinity for the heart, reducing palpitations and the fear that often accompanies them. This is discussed in depth in *Successful Stress Control* by David Hoffmann. Recent advances in the field of neurology have come about through the examination of claims for herbal remedies. Concerning therapy of nerve tissue as such, we can consider two examples, the use of ginkgo for a range of conditions which include Alzheimer's disease, and feverfew in the treatment of migraine.

Alzheimer's Disease

Once thought rare, this neurological disorder of the brain is now considered the largest single cause of senile dementia. Although no chemical cure exists, great attention is being given to the oriental remedy ginkgo leaf in the treatment of this problem. Much of the clinical and pharmacological research comes from France and Germany, where the herb has a reputation as an antimicrobial. Recent clinical research showed profound activity on brain function and cerebral circulation. It is effective in patients with vascular disorders, in all types of dementia and even in patients suffering from cognitive disorders secondary to depression. Of special concern are people who are just beginning to experience such problems; for them, ginkgo may delay deterioration and enable them to maintain a normal life. It is quite safe, even in doses many times higher than those usually recommended.[4] Ginkgo is best taken regularly over a long period of time. A good dosage regime would be a 40-milligram tablet taken three times a day.

Migraine

Feverfew is a remedy well known to medical herbalists which is now being used by orthodox medicine. Used throughout medical history as a bitter tonic and remedy for severe headaches, it has recently gained a reputation as a "cure" for migraine. Clinicians at the London Migraine Clinic observed that patients were improving when taking the herb. Luckily these doctors had the inquiring and open minds of true scientists and so started their own investigations, and their observations were soon reported in the medical journals. Plant constituents called sesquiterpene lactones may inhibit the prostaglandins and histamine released during inflammation. This prevents the spasming of blood vessels in the brain that causes the pain.

There are a number of ways to use feverfew to treat migraine safely. Eating a fresh leaf every day, possibly between bread, is effective. If no fresh plant is available, take 50 to 100 milligrams in tablet form daily.

The action of feverfew will be aided by drinking an infusion of equal parts of chamomile and hawthorn. This combination will promote relaxation, dilate blood vessels and ease any tendency to nausea. Rosemary or lavender oil rubbed into the temples may ease an attack. Any predisposing trigger must be identified by a skilled practitioner; these can be dietary, stress-related, postural or hormonal.

Stress and Anxiety

Nervines offer a range of ways to relax, uplift or put to sleep an overworked mind and body. Our medicine chest has chamomile, linden flower and valerian. Essential oils used in massage or added to the bath will relax in a wonderful way. For stress we have the adaptogen Siberian ginseng.

No matter what the stress is, the body responds in the same physiological way. It might be illness, overwork, a heat wave or falling in love—the response is the same. It is called the general adaptation syndrome, and it is this that adaptogens help. To help deal with any stress, take Siberian ginseng daily and use chamomile, linden flower or valerian as needed for relaxation. For short-term stress use 1 gram of Siberian ginseng a day for up to a month, or 250-500 milligrams over longer periods.

Insomnia

Sleeping pills cause more problems than they solve, and are addictive and well worth avoiding. Herbs offer a safe and effective alternative. An infusion of chamomile flowers made with one teaspoonful to a cup of boiling water is often sufficient. This may be made stronger if needed. Linden flowers can be used at the same dosage and are especially valuable for people with blood pressure problems. A stronger remedy is valerian. This has an unusual taste and may be taken as a tablet or tincture about half an hour before going to bed. A herb bath is very relaxing. Fill a muslin bag with chamomile, linden flowers or lavender and hang it from the faucet so that the hot water runs through it. Don't fall asleep in the bath!

Skin Problems

As the largest organ of the body, the skin plays a vital role in health and wholeness. It protects, is an organ of elimination, helps control body temperature and is a sensory organ. Problems of the skin can be expressions of whole-body conditions. Most of the herbs in the medicine chest can play a useful role in treating skin problems.

Eczema: This is best treated internally, as the cause is usually a constitutional one. The alterative remedies are specific. From the medicine chest we have nettles and echinacea, but in addition consider cleavers, yellow dock or red clover. The cleansing action of these alteratives will be aided by combining them with a relaxing nervine such as chamomile, linden flowers or valerian. If under stress, the adrenals can be supported with the adaptogen Siberian ginseng. A possible combination would be equal parts nettles and chamomile as an infusion taken 3 times a day. Add 1 teaspoonful of the combination to a cup of hot water and steep for 5 to 10 minutes. There are many external treatments for the skin and the most effective will vary from person to person. Essential oil of lavender or chamomile mixed with almond oil or an aqueous cream is very cooling. A compress or poultice using plaintain or chickweed will reduce irritation.

Cold Sores: This common manifestation of the herpes virus is usually an expression of lowered body resistance. Herbs that strengthen resistance and immune response should be taken internally. Echinacea and Siberian ginseng should be used to boost immunity, combined with nettles and golden seal. Externally, apply dilute tincture of golden seal or calendula.

Boils: Local infections of the skin should be treated internally with antimicrobials such as echinacea, combined with a cleansing alterative such as nettles. A decoction of equal parts of these two herbs drunk three times a day will help; so will eating raw garlic. A hot poultice will help draw the boil.

Wounds and Abrasions: Bathe the cut with an infusion of calendula; a diluted tincture will also do. Applying distilled witch hazel will stop bleeding and promote healing. Golden seal will speed healing, applied as a powder or salve.

REMEDIES FOR THE MEDICINE CHEST

In a book of this small size it is impossible to give the remedies the full attention they deserve, but let's focus on chamomile to suggest the possibilities, and deal with the others more briefly.

CHAMOMILE *Matricaria chamomilla*

Chamomile has been part of herbal medicine for as long as records exist, and is still very much present in health care, being used wherever it grows in the world. Its medical uses include insomnia, anxiety, menopausal depression, loss of appetite, dyspepsia, diarrhea, colic, aches and pains of flu, migraine, neuralgia, teething, vertigo, motion sickness, conjunctivitis, inflamed skin, and urticaria.

Chamomile is the most widely used relaxing nervine herb in the western world. Relaxing the nervous system, it is especially valuable when anxiety and tension produce digestive problems. It makes a wonderful late night tea, ensuring restful sleep. In Europe it is used for anxious children or teething infants, by simply adding the tea to a bath. As an antispasmodic herb, it relaxes peripheral nerves and muscles, easing cramps. When the body is at ease, peace of mind and heart follows. Rich in aromatic essential oil, it acts on the digestive system, gently promoting proper function, soothing the walls of the intestines, easing griping pains and helping the removal of gas. Chamomile tea relieves indigestion, calming inflammations such as gastritis and helping prevent ulcer formation. Using the essential oil as a steam inhalation allows the oils to reach inflamed membranes in the sinuses and lungs. Its gentle antimicrobial action helps the body resist pathogenic microorganisms. As an anticatarrhal it helps remove catarrhal buildup from the sinus and so is used for colds and allergies such as hayfever.

There is a wealth of information on its biochemical components, but this does not tell us much about the benefits of the herb in healing. The activity of a whole plant is always more than the sum of its parts, just as a person is more than the sum of his biochemistry. Herbal medicine treats the unique individual and not just the manifest disease. Herbs can be very powerful in addressing symptomatology, but we limit their potential if we stay at this level. Knowing the chemistry of sesquiterpenes is not the same as knowing chamomile!

The herb may be used in all the ways plants can be prepared as medicines. Used fresh or dried, it should be infused to make tea. The tincture is an excellent way of ensuring all the plant's components are extracted and available for the body. In aromatherapy the essential oil of chamomile is a valued preparation.

Dosage: Dried herb: an infusion of 1 teaspoonful drunk as needed. Tablets: 250 milligrams taken 1-3 a day, or 500 milligrams taken before bedtime. (Best standardized on apigenin.)

BONESET *Eupatorium perfoliatum*

Actions: Diaphoretic, aperient, antispasmodic, diuretic, anticatarrhal, bitter. Boneset eases symptoms associated with influenza and other infections that feel "fluish." It does not rid the body of the virus, but it does make the whole experience more bearable by relieving the aches and pains. It may be used as symptomatic relief in muscular rheumatism. As a good diaphoretic it helps the body deal with any associated fever.[5] It is effective in clearing sinus catarrh. Additionally, its mild aperient, bitter and diuretic actions make boneset a good general cleansing remedy.

Dosage: Dried herb: an infusion of 1 teaspoonful drunk hot three times a day. Tablets: 250 milligrams taken twice a day.

CALENDULA (Marigold) *Calendula officinalis*

Actions: Anti-inflammatory, astringent, vulnerary, antifungal, cholagogue, emmenagogue.

A beautiful flower long used throughout Europe for wound healing and ulcer treatments. Part of its healing power appears to be based on the presence of biochemicals called terpenes. A triterpene glycoside called calenduloside B exerts a marked anti-ulcerous and sedative action. Researchers say this chemical is devoid of any irritating properties and is of insignificant toxicity.[6] If this is the case with an extracted constituent, much more can be expected from the whole plant! Ideal for treating local skin problems, it may be used safely for inflammations on the skin, whether due to infection or physical damage. For any external bleeding or wound, bruising, strains, as well as in slow-healing wounds and skin ulcers. It is an ideal first aid treatment of minor burns. Local treatments may be with a lotion, a poultice or compress. Internally it is used for digestive inflammations or ulceration. As a hepatic, it aids treatment of gallbladder problems and can help in many of the vague digestive complaints that are called indigestion. Calendula has antifungal activity and may be used both internally and externally to combat such infections. It is a normalizer of the menstrual process.

Dosage: Dried herb: an infusion of 1 teaspoonful drunk three times a day. Tablets: 250 milligrams taken twice a day. (Best standardized on saponins.)

DANDELION *Taraxacum officinalis*
Actions: Bitter tonic, hepatic, diuretic, alterative.
The root is a bitter tonic for the liver, stimulating the activity of both liver and gallbladder. This increases the flow of bile, helping in constipation and indigestion. The leaves are powerful diuretics, and although comparable to drug diuretics, the herb does not leach potassium from the body. This combination of liver and kidney effects make it a good cleansing remedy in skin and rheumatic problems.

Dosage: Dried herb: an infusion of 1 teaspoonful drunk twice a day. Tablets: 400 milligrams taken two or three times a day. (Best standardized on potassium.)

DEVIL'S CLAW *Harpagophytum procumbens*
Actions: Anti-inflammatory, analgesic.
This is a remedy from the Kalahari Desert in Namibia with a well-deserved reputation as a rheumatic remedy. A group of glycosides called harpagosides found in the root show a striking anti-inflammatory effect in joints.[7] An effective treatment in some cases of arthritis, it helps most where there is marked inflammation and pain associated with the arthritis.

Dosage: Dried herb: a decoction of 1 teaspoonful drunk three times a day. Tablets: 150 milligrams taken three times a day before meals. (Best standardized on harpagosides.)

ECHINACEA *Echinacea purpurea*
Actions: Antimicrobial, alterative.

Echinacea is the prime remedy to help the body rid itself of microbial infections. Immunity is helped via a stimulation of white blood cell production[8] and a polysaccharide that is antiviral.[9] Effective against both bacterial and viral attacks, it may be used in conjunction with other herbs for infection anywhere in the body. For example, in combination with uva-ursi it effectively treats cystitis. It is especially useful for infections of the upper respiratory tract such as laryngitis and tonsillitis, and for catarrhal conditions of the nose and sinus. As a mouthwash, it speeds the treatment of pyorrhea and gingivitis. It may be used as an external lotion for septic sores and cuts.

Dosage: Dried herb: a decoction of 1 teaspoonful drunk three times a day. Tablets: 50 milligrams taken twice a day for long-term use, or 1 tablet every 2 hours for acute problems. Possibly the best form is the preserved fresh juice; take 20 drops in liquid 3 times a day or every 2 hours in acute problems.

ELECAMPANE *Inula helenium*
Actions: Expectorant, diaphoretic, antimicrobial.

This beautiful herb has been traditionally used in the treatment of tuberculosis, a use supported by modern research on the lactones it contains.[10] An effective remedy for bronchitis and asthma, or as a tonic support for the lungs in general, it is safe for children as well as the elderly. A herb to consider if you live in a smoggy environment.

Dosage: Dried herb: an infusion of 1 teaspoonful drunk as hot as possible twice a day. Tablets: 250 milligrams taken twice a day.

FEVERFEW *Tanacetum parthenium*
Actions: Anti-inflammatory, vasodilatory, relaxant, digestive bitter, uterine stimulant.

Feverfew has regained its deserved reputation as a primary remedy in the treatment and prevention of migraine headaches, especially those that are relieved by applying warmth to the head.[11] It may also help arthritis in the painfully active inflammatory stage. Dizziness and tinnitus may be eased, especially if it is used in conjunction with other remedies. Feverfew will relieve painful periods and sluggish menstrual flow.

Dosage: Dried herb: an infusion of 1 teaspoonful drunk once a day. Tablets: 50 to 100 milligrams of freeze-dried plant taken twice a day with food.

GINKGO *Ginkgo biloba*
Actions: Antimicrobial, vasodilator.

Traditionally known as an antimicrobial and antitubercular agent, new research has shown a profound effect for ginkgo on brain function and

cerebral circulation.[12] A safe remedy that helps in peripheral circulatory problems of the arms, hands, legs and feet, it is effective in people with vascular disorders and in all types of dementia. It is of special importance to people who are just beginning to experience cognitive deterioration. Ginkgo extract delays further deterioration, enabling such people to maintain normal lives. It offers much for the treatment of short-term memory deficit, and many problems of the elderly, including Alzheimer's disease. Ginkgo is quite safe, even in doses many times higher than those usually recommended.
Dosage: Dried herb: an infusion of 1 teaspoonful drunk twice a day. Tablets: 40 milligrams taken three times a day. (Best standardized on ginkgo flavonglycoside.)

GOLDEN SEAL *Hydrastis canadensis*
Actions: Tonic, astringent, anticatarrhal, antimicrobial, laxative, uterine stimulant, bitter.
One of our most useful remedies, owing much of its value to the tonic effects it has on the mucous membranes of the body. This is why it is of such help in all digestive problems, from peptic ulcers to colitis. Its bitter stimulation helps reverse loss of appetite, and the alkaloids it contains stimulate bile production and secretion. All catarrhal conditions improve with golden seal, especially sinus ones. Traditionally it has been used during labor to help contractions, but it is for just this reason that it should be avoided during pregnancy. Applied externally, it can be helpful in eczema, ringworm, itching, earache and conjunctivitis.
Dosage: Dried herb: a decoction of a half-teaspoonful drunk twice a day. Tablets: 250 milligrams taken twice a day for not longer than two months. (Best standardized on alkaloids.)

HAWTHORN *Crataegus oxyacantha*
Actions: Cardiac tonic, hypotensive.
Hawthorn provides us with a tonic remedy for the heart and circulatory system. It acts in a normalizing way upon the heart by either stimulating or depressing its activity, depending upon the need. It has the vital property of dilating the coronary arteries, and so increasing oxygen availability to the heart.[13] As a long-term treatment, it is safe to use in heart failure or weakness, and in cases of palpitations. As a tonic for the circulatory system, its main use is in the treatment of high blood pressure, arteriosclerosis and angina pectoris.
Dosage: Dried herb: an infusion of 1 teaspoonful drunk twice a day. Tablets: 250 milligrams taken twice a day. (Best standardized on flavonoids.)

LINDEN FLOWER *Tilia europaea*
Actions: Nervine, antispasmodic, hypotensive, diaphoretic, diuretic.
A safe and widely applicable relaxing herb for anxiety and tension, it is also

used in Europe to prevent and treat arteriosclerosis and hypertension. This makes it a specific in cases of elevated blood pressure associated with nervous tension. It will help any condition that is worsened through stress. A good relaxing nervine for children. As a diaphoretic it helps in feverish problems.
Dosage: Dried herb: an infusion of 1 teaspoonful drunk twice a day. Tablets: 250 milligrams taken twice a day. (Best standardized on flavonoids.)

MARSHMALLOW *Althaea officinalis*
Actions: Root: demulcent, diuretic, emollient, vulnerary. Leaf: demulcent, expectorant, diuretic, emollient.
The high mucilage content of marshmallow makes it an excellent demulcent that can be used whenever needed.[14] The root is used primarily for digestive problems and on the skin, and the leaf for the lungs and the urinary system. In all inflammations of the digestive tract, such as those of the mouth, gastritis, peptic ulcer, enteritis and colitis, the root is best. For bronchitis, respiratory catarrh and irritating coughs, the leaves should be considered. It is also soothing in cases of urethritis and urinary gravel—in fact, it soothes mucous membrane anywhere. Externally, the root is used in varicose veins and ulcers, as well as abscesses and boils.

MEADOWSWEET *Filipendula ulmaria*
Actions: Anti-inflammatory, carminative, antacid, anti-emetic, astringent, diuretic.
A wonderful remedy for digestive problems, rheumatism and arthritis. It soothes the whole of the digestive tract, reducing stomach acidity, easing the discomfort of gastritis and ulceration. As meadowsweet was the herb that aspirin was first made from, it contains safe aspirin-like anti-inflammatories. The other actions of the herb ensure that there is no danger of damaging the stomach in the way that the drug does.
Dosage: Dried herb: an infusion of 1 teaspoonful drunk twice a day. Tablets: 250 milligrams taken twice a day. (Best standardized on salicylates.)

MILK THISTLE *Silybum marianum*
Actions: Hepatic, galactogogue, demulcent.
As its name implies, it promotes milk secretion and is perfectly safe to be used by all breast-feeding mothers. Milk thistle can also be used to increase the secretion and flow of bile from the liver and gallbladder. Its traditional use as a liver tonic has been supported by research showing that a constituent called silymarin protects liver cells from chemical damage.[15] It is used in a whole range of liver and gallbladder conditions including hepatitis and cirrhosis.

Dosage: Dried herb: an infusion of 1 teaspoon drunk twice a day. Tablets: 100 milligrams taken three times a day. (Best standardized on silymarin.)

NETTLES *Urtica dioica*
Actions: Tonic, alterative, astringent.
An invaluable source of vitamins and minerals, making a good spring tonic. An excellent treatment for anemia, they are rich in iron and the vitamin C that helps its assimilation. Nettles increase excretion of uric acid, so helping arthritis and gout. Applied to the skin they reduce arthritic swelling (effective but brave!). As an astringent they will reduce bleeding and diarrhea. A good general tonic for eczema.
Dosage: Dried herb: an infusion of 1 teaspoonful drunk twice a day. Tablets: 260 milligrams taken twice a day.

ST. JOHN'S WORT *Hypericum perforatum*
Actions: Anti-inflammatory, astringent, vulnerary, nervine.
A remedy with an ancient reputation as a healer for the nerves. It is used for pain and stress related problems such as neuralgia. A specific for menopausal changes that trigger irritability and anxiety, it will also ease the pain of fibrositis and rheumatism. On the skin it speeds wound healing and reduces inflammation. Exciting new research has found that constituents called hypericin and pseudohypericin combat retrovirus infections. This is the group that includes the acquired immunodeficiency syndrome (AIDS) virus, so this discovery presents exciting possibilities.[16]
Dosage: Dried herb: an infusion of 1 teaspoonful drunk twice a day. Tablets: 250 milligrams taken twice a day. (Best standardized on hypericin.)

SIBERIAN GINSENG *Eleutherococcus senticosus*
Actions: Adaptogen, a circulatory stimulant, vasodilator.
This herb may be safely used to increase stamina in the face of undue demands and stress. These may be physical or mental—they are the same to the body. It is used for debility, exhaustion and depression, except where these are due to a specific medical condition that calls for defined treatment. It has a growing reputation for increasing all kinds of body resistance.
Dosage: For short-term stress use 1 gram of Siberian ginseng a day for up to a month, or 250-500 milligrams over longer periods. (Best standardized on eleutherosides.)

UVA-URSI *Arctostaphylos uva-ursi*
Actions: Diuretic, antimicrobial, astringent.
An effective treatment for cystitis, this oil-rich leaf may be used in an infection of the urinary system.[17] It will soothe associated inflammation in the bladder and other areas, and will help in the treatment of kidney stones and gravel. Uva-ursi makes a good general diuretic.

Dosage: Dried herb: an infusion of 1 teaspoonful drunk twice a day. Tablets: 1000 milligrams taken three times a day. (Best standardized on arbutin.)

    VALERIAN   *Valeriana officinalis*
Actions: Sedative, antispasmodic, hypotensive, carminative.
Valerian is one of the most useful relaxing nervines that is available to us. This fact is recognized by orthodox medicine, as is shown by its inclusion in many pharmacopoeias as a sedative. It may safely be used to reduce tension and anxiety, overexcitability and hysterical states.[18] It is an effective aid in insomnia, producing a natural healing sleep. As an antispasmodic herb, it will aid in the relief of cramp and intestinal colic and will also be useful for the cramps and pain of periods. As a pain-reliever it is most indicated when pain is associated with tension. Valerian can help in migraine and rheumatic pain.
Dosage: Dried herb: an infusion of 1 teaspoonful drunk twice a day. Tablets: 400 milligrams taken twice a day, or 800 milligrams taken before bedtime. (Best standardized on valerenic acid.)

Healing Remedies from the Kitchen

Food is the best medicine, for it is from our nutrition that we nurture the life in us. Herbal remedies are simply a specific variety of vegetables! Ones that would not sell too well in supermarkets, but are a vital part of nature's garden. The healing potential of the herbs and spices found in most kitchens is surprising. Much first aid and treatment of common problems can be undertaken with these remedies. There is not the space to review their uses, as excellent guides to their medicinal uses have been written.[19] As an example of the potential, consider garlic.

    GARLIC   *Allium sativum*
Actions: Antiseptic, antiviral, diaphoretic, cholagogue, hypotensive, antispasmodic.
Garlic is among the few herbs that are universally used and recognized. It is one of the most effective antimicrobial plants available.[20] As the volatile oil is secreted largely via the lungs, it is used in infections such as chronic bronchitis, respiratory catarrh, recurrent colds and influenza. It is used as a preventive for infectious conditions in general. For the digestive tract it has been found that garlic will help natural bacterial flora while killing pathogenic organisms. It has been used externally for the treatment of ringworm and threadworm. Garlic has an international reputation for lowering both blood pressure and blood cholesterol levels and for generally improving the health of the cardiovascular system.
Dosage: Fresh raw bulb garlic: 1 clove a day. Capsules (or "perles"): 2 capsules three times a day, *with food.*

Other culinary herbs of note for health care are:

Marjoram, rosemary, oregano, basil, thyme, sage, fennel, dill, aniseed, celery seed, cinnamon, cayenne, mustard, ginger, horseradish, tea, coffee

THE PREPARATION OF HERBS

Part of the art of herbal medicine is knowing what techniques to use in preparing the remedies. Methods have been developed over the centuries to enable their properties to be released. After the right choice of herbs has been made, the best way to prepare them must be selected, choosing which process will release the biochemical constituents needed for healing without insulting the integrity of the plant by isolating fractions of the whole. The property of any herb is not just the sum of the actions of the various chemicals present. There is a synergy at work that acts to create a therapeutic whole that is more than the sum of its parts. If the method of preparation destroys or loses part of the whole, much of the healing power is lost.

The art and science of herbal medicine making are beyond the range of this book. It is a fascinating and enjoyable field, with many excellent books describing the techniques that can be used at home.[21,22] Here we shall only describe the preparations mentioned in this book.

Infusion

If you know how to make tea, you know how to make an infusion. It is the simplest method of using herbs, and both fresh or dried herbs may be used. Note that where one part of dried herb is prescribed, it can be replaced with three parts of the fresh herb, the difference being due to the higher water content of the fresh herb. Therefore, if the instructions call for one teaspoonful of dried herb, three teaspoons of fresh herb can be substituted.

To make an infusion:

• Take a china or glass teapot which has been warmed and put one teaspoonful of the dried herb or herb mixture into it for each cup of tea.

• Pour a cup of boiling water in for each teaspoonful of herb that is already in the pot and then put the lid on. Leave to steep for ten to fifteen minutes. Infusions may be drunk hot—preferable for a medicinal herb tea—or cold. They may be sweetened with licorice root, honey or brown sugar.

Herbal teabags can be made by filling muslin bags with herbal mixtures, taking care to remember how many teaspoonfuls have been put into each bag. They can be used in the same way as ordinary teabags.

To make larger quantities to last for a while, the proportion should be one ounce of herb to one pint of water; store in a refrigerator. The shelf life is not very long, as the infusion is so full of life force that any microorganism that enters it will thrive. If there is any sign of fermentation, the infusion should be discarded. Ideally infusions should be prepared fresh for each use.

Infusions are best for leaves, flowers or green stems, in which the substances wanted are easily accessible. To infuse bark, root or seeds, it is best to powder them first to break down some of their cell walls and make them more water-accessible. Seeds, such as fennel or aniseed, should be slightly bruised before infusing to release the volatile oils from the cells. Aromatic herbs should be infused in a pot with a well-sealing lid, ensuring only a minimum loss of volatile oil through evaporation.

With heat-sensitive herbs (because of volatile oils or their constituents breakdown at high temperature), make a cold infusion. The proportion of herb to water is the same, but in this case the infusion should be left for six to twelve hours in a well-sealed earthenware pot.

Apart from their medicinal use, herbs make an exquisite addition to life and can open a whole world of subtle delights and pleasures. They are not only medicines or alternatives to coffee, but make excellent teas in their own right.

Decoction

Whenever the herb to be used is hard and woody, it is best to make a decoction rather than an infusion to ensure that the soluble contents of the herb actually reach the water. Roots, rhizomes, wood, bark, nuts and some seeds are hard and their cell walls are very strong, so more heat is needed than for infusions—the herb has to be boiled in the water.

To make a decoction:

- Put one teaspoonful of dried herb or three teaspoonfuls of fresh material for each cup of water into a pot or saucepan. Dried herbs should be powdered or broken into small pieces, while fresh material should be cut into small pieces. If large quantities are made, use one ounce of dried herb for each pint of water. The container should be glass, ceramic or earthenware. If metal, it should be enameled. Never use aluminum.
- Add the appropriate amount of water to the herbs.
- Bring to a boil and simmer for the time given for the mixture or specific herb, usually ten to fifteen minutes. If the herb contains volatile oils, put a lid on.
- Strain the tea while it is still hot.

A decoction can be used in the same way as an infusion. If you are making up a remedy containing both soft and woody herbs, it is best to prepare an infusion and a decoction separately, to ensure that the more sensitive herbs are treated appropriately. When using a woody herb that contains a lot of volatile oils, such as valerian root, it is best to powder it as finely as possible and then use it in an infusion, so that the oils do not boil away.

Compress
This is an excellent way of applying a remedy to the skin. Soak a clean linen or cotton cloth in a hot herbal tea and apply it to the affected part of the body. Use as hot as can be tolerated, and cover with a towel to hold in the heat. When cool replace with another. For a cold compress, use the same method but simply let the tea cool.

Poultice
This more therapeutically active method uses fresh or dried plant rather than a liquid form. Mash or crush fresh plant material and either heat over boiling water or mix with a small amount of boiling water to make a paste. Apply directly to the skin as hot as possible, and hold it in place with gauze. Powder dried herb and mix with hot water to create a paste. If using stimulating herbs such as mustard, apply them between two layers of cloth.

HERBAL NEXT STEPS

If this little booklet has whetted your appetite and you would like to explore further, here are some suggestions:

- Visit nature. Spend time in natural wild places, and experience yourself as being truly part of our world.
- Get to know the herbs. Learn to identify them, know where they live and grow.
- Grow the herbs. This may be in a garden or little pots!
- Use them for healing but also as an enhancement of life. Make cosmetics, flower wreaths, cook with them, etc. You will be surprised at the ways in which herbs can be part of your life.
- Further education in herbalism. Herbalism in the USA is in the paradoxical position of experiencing a flowering of interest in all its aspects, yet lacking educational avenues to explore. This is one of the very few developed countries where medical herbalism is not legally recognized, making professional training a challenge!

As there is no licensing body, no degree-giving schools of herbalism currently exist. Naturopathic medicine covers the basics within the context of their broad approach, as do the acupuncture colleges for Oriental herbalism. The National College of Naturopathic Medicine in Portland, Oregon and John Bastyr College in Seattle, Washington have the best "botanic" medicine courses.

The best herbal education is offered by schools that are educationally unorthodox. Such places have developed where herbalists live, rather than where the demand is! They are small scale and on the whole excellent. As they are expressions of the vision, skills and wisdom of the herbalists involved, they have their unique strengths and weaknesses. Some offer full training, others are based on workshop formats or correspondence courses. For a comprehensive listing of such schools, please contact the California School of Herbal Studies, P.O. Box 39, Forestville, CA 95436, (707) 887-7457. The School offers courses that range from the practical skills of gardening, wildcrafting and medicine making to herbal therapeutics for both the beginner and health care professionals.

BIBLIOGRAPHY

There is an ever-growing number of books relating to herbalism. Here is a partial selection.

Bremness, Leslie. *The Complete Book of Herbs.* New York: Viking Studio Books 1988.

Grieve, Mrs. M. *A Modern Herbal,* volumes I and II. New York: Dover Publications, 1971.

Hoffmann, David. *The Herbal Handbook.* Richmond, Vermont: Inner Traditions, 1989.

Hoffmann, David. *The Holistic Herbal.* Salisbury, Dorset, U.K.: Element Books, 1983.

Hoffmann, David. *Successful Stress Control.* Richmond, Vermont: Inner Traditions, 1986.

Mabey, Richard. *The New Age Herbalist.* New York: Collier Books, 1988.

Mills, Simon. *Dictionary of Modern Herbalism.* Wellingborough, Northants, U.K.: Thorsons, 1987.

Stuart, Malcom, ed. *Color Dictionary of Herbs and Herbalism.* New York: Van Notrand, 1979.

Thomson, William. *Medicines From the Earth.* New York: McGraw-Hill, 1978.

REFERENCES

1. Bland, J. *Intestinal Toxicity and Inner Cleansing.* New Canaan, Connecticut: Keats Publishing, 1987.
2. Ibid.
3. Hahn et al. On the pharmacology and toxicology of silymarin, an anti-hepatotoxic active principle from *Silybum marianum* (L.) Gaertn. *Arzneitmittel. Forschung.* (Jun 68) 18(6):698–704.
4. Warburton, D.M. Clinical psychopharmacology of *Ginkgo biloba* extract. *Presse Med.* 1986 Sep 25; 15(31):1595–604.
5. Claus, E.P., *Pharmacognosy,* 4th ed. Philadelphia: Lea & Febiger, 1961.
6. Iatsyno et al. Pharmacology of calenduloside B, a new triterpene glycoside from the roots of Calendula officinalis. *Farmakol. Toksikol.* 41(5):556–60, 1978.
7. Eichler et al. Antiphlogistic, analgesic and spasmolytic effect of harpagoside, a glycoside from the root of *Harpagophytum procumbens. Arzneitmittel. Forschung.* 20(1):107–9 1970.
8. Kuhn O. *Arzneitmittel Forschung.* 2,467, 1952.
9. Wacker and Hilbig. *Planta Medica* 33, 89–102. 1978.
10. *Chemical Abstracts* 87, 167–217, 1977.
11. Johnson, Kadam, Hylands and Hylands. Efficacy of feverfew as prophylactic treatment of migraine. *British Medical Journal* 291(6495):569–73, 1985.
12. Bensky and Gamble. *Chinese Herbal Medicine.* Eastland Press, 1986.
13. Ammon and Handel. *Planta Medica* 43:209, 1981.
14. Delaveau et al. *Planta Medica* 40:49, 1980.
15. Hahn, Lehmann, Kurten, Uebel and Vogel. On the pharmacology and toxicology of silymarin, an antihepatotoxic active principle from *Silybum marianum. Arzneitmittel. Forschung.* 18(6):698–704 1968.
16. Meruelo, Lavie and Lavie. Therapeutic agents with dramatic antiretroviral activity and little toxity at effective doses. *Proc. Natl. Acad. Sci.* 85:5230–5234, 1988.
17. Martindale. *Extra Pharmacopeia* 26th ed.
18. Hendriks et al. *Planta Medica* 45:150, 1982.
19. Heinerman, J. *The Complete Book of Spices.* New Canaan, Connecticut: Keats Publishing, 1983.
20. Hoffmann, D.L. *The Holistic Herbal.* Salisbury, Dorset, U.K.: Element Books, 1988.
21. Bremness, L. *The Complete Book of Herbs.* New York: Viking Studio Books, 1988.